50 THINGS TO KNOW ABOUT BACHELORS DEGREE IN PUBLIC POLICY AND HEALTH

I0506787

50 THINGS TO KNOW BOOK SERIES REVIEWS FROM READERS

I recently downloaded a couple of books from this series to read over the weekend thinking I would read just one or two. However, I so loved the books that I read all the six books I had downloaded in one go and ended up downloading a few more today. Written by different authors, the books offer practical advice on how you can perform or achieve certain goals in life, which in this case is how to have a better life.

The information is simple to digest and learn from, and is incredibly useful. There are also resources listed at the end of the book that you can use to get more information.

50 Things To Know To Have A Better Life: Self-Improvement Made Easy!

Author Dannii Cohen

This book is very helpful and provides simple tips on how to improve your everyday life. I found it to be useful in improving my overall attitude.

50 Things to Know For Your Mindfulness & Meditation Journey
Author Nina Edmondso

Quick read with 50 short and easy tips for what to think about before starting to homeschool.

50 Things to Know About Getting Started with Homeschool by Author Amanda Walton

I really enjoyed the voice of the narrator, she speaks in a soothing tone. The book is a really great reminder of things we might have known we could do during stressful times, but forgot over the years.

Author Harmony Hawaii

There is so much waste in our society today. Everyone should be forced to read this book. I know I am passing it on to my family.

50 Things to Know to Downsize Your Life: How To Downsize, Organize, And Get Back to Basics

Author Lisa Rusczyk Ed. D.

Great book to get you motivated and understand why you may be losing motivation. Great for that person who wants to start getting healthy, or just for you when you need motivation while having an established workout routine.

50 Things To Know To Stick With A Workout: Motivational Tips To Start The New You Today

Author Sarah Hughes

50 THINGS TO KNOW ABOUT GETTING A BACHELOR'S DEGREE IN PUBLIC HEALTH POLICY

Reflections From a Public Health Policy Major

Mary S. Kim

Cover designed by: Ivana Stamenkovic
Cover Image: https://pixabay.com/photos/student-library-books-book-learn-3500990/

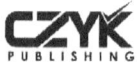

CZYK Publishing Since 2011.
50 Things to Know

Lock Haven, PA
All rights reserved.
ISBN: 9798597881119

ABOUT THE AUTHOR

My name is Mary Kim (but you probably know that by now already!). I attended the University of California, Irvine (UCI) and entered as Undeclared. The daunting major of "Unknown…"

Like so many high school graduates, I aimlessly wandered into the phase of applying to colleges with no clear understanding of how majors worked and even how each college offered different majors! I know that so many of you go into college so confused on how to make a decision that could really influence your entire life. As I wandered the first year at UCI, I slowly found my calling in Public Health, but it wasn't an easy one. College majors are hard to choose, and I hope that I can shed some light on one of the bajillion majors that college has to offer.

INTRODUCTION

*"Consistency of effort over the long run is **everything**."*

Angela Duckworth

Different majors at universities are always the most daunting task when applying to colleges. Often times, this confusion arises from the lack of preparation in high school when it comes to college majors and the routes that should be taken in order to pursue certain careers. Time and time again, students enter into the college world with little to no education in regard to what their major actually pertains to or the number of other majors that are offered at their university. There are so many other majors that colleges have to offer that many students are unaware about as a result of simple misinformation translated over when applying to colleges. These lowkey majors offer much opportunity for professional growth as well as income wise. The major of Public Health is one of those majors. A major in Public Health opens the door to so many opportunities yet this major does not get as much attention as some other majors do. For this reason, I would like to present with you some facts on the major itself and ways to succeed when pursuing a Public Health degree (or just a college degree for that matter). From one once inexperienced college graduate, take these words of advice and ponder on them as college really has so much more to offer than many think!

(PUBLIC HEALTH CAREER ROUTES)

1. PHARMACEUTICALS

Although there is much controversy on the big pharma world and the Public Health world, there is no doubt that there are much professional growth opportunities in the world of pharmaceuticals. Whether that is you want to go into sales or marketing, a Public Health major can get you right into the world of pharmaceutical sales or marketing. Public Health is a great major choice for individuals looking to go into the medical world but on the business side of things!

2. HOSPITAL ADMINISTRATOR

Being a Hospital Administrator opens the door to so many opportunities in a Hospital. A Hospital is essentially a business. Within that business, to ensure that everything runs smoothly, a person with a business mind is needed to handle departmental activities! This deals with planning for the hospital in terms of public relations, community events and creating and maintaining policies within the hospital

3. DOCTOR

A Public Health major is a great route to go if you are unsure on what kind of PHD or MD program that you want to go into, for example. Public Health opens up the door and potential for pre-med students if they're still unsure on exactly what medical degree that they want but know that they DO want a medical degree post college. The courses in Public Health can also fill as pre-requisites for medical schools, but that's something you'd want to look up depending on your university & the medical school that you want to apply to!

4. CENTER FOR DISEASE CONTROL AND PREVENTION (CDC)

Now, this is an absolute given when it comes to Public Health as a major. The obvious path to go down with this major is written all over the actual name of the major itself! If you are interested in working in the CDC, Public Health is a great road for that! Not only do you learn community strategies and disease control outreach and so much more in Public Health, but with this, you could work for a world-renowned organization to make a real difference

5. EPIDEMIOLOGIST

Not too many people know what an Epidemiologist is, and I will admit, neither did I! This is an awesome route to go if you are into Statistics and are just a major observer in general. An Epidemiologist focuses on the pattern of disease within a community (or the world if there's a pandemic) and observes the patterns and irregularities. An Epidemiologist is a great profession to go in to as it aims to really bring to light disparities in communities and certain groups of people that are of less advantage

6. MEDICAL WORLD MARKETING

Now, it's getting interesting…. Are you wondering how in the world does Public Health relate to

Marketing?! Well, that's actually my position right now! Public Health is such a neat major as it gets you into the "medical world" playing field, without you necessarily having to fully commit to becoming a Doctor of some sort. I knew I wanted to be in the demanding medical world force, but I didn't want to become a Doctor or a Physician's Assistant (another good profession Public Health opens the doors to) so I went the business route with Public Health!

7. RESEARCHER

As this job title is extremely broad, it's meant to be that way! Public Health allows for individuals with the degree to take a leap into different positions to pursue Research as many professionals know the importance of having a Public Health major on board their team. In this day and age, as Public Health continues to become a growing profession, a valuable member of the team with a Public Health background can offer analysis' on things that others may not be able to see

8. COMMUNITY OUTREACH PROGRAMMER

Raising the awareness within communities is of utmost importance and it took me throughout college to realize that. Health disparities are absolutely real and none of it is really apparent! It's important to spread awareness to groups of people that are less likely to have that information accessible to them. If you like helping people and have always loved to give back, Public Health is a great route for you to adventure on

9. PUBLIC HEALTH ATTORNEY

Strange, right?! But yet again, the Public Health major strikes back with more unique, yet random, BUT a high-paying job! Although additional education is required post-college, this profession is focused entirely on a simple phrase, "how can we better our community through public health policies and regulations." Although if you think about it, Public Health really is in its entirety focused around that phrase, but being a Lawyer makes all the difference because then you can actually pass those policies and regulations!

10. PROFESSOR

With a Public Health degree, there are many opportunities to enter the world of education such as being a professor at a university! If you have an interest in Public Health, but also would love to become a professor of some sorts later along the road, then this major would be perfect for you. There are many courses that are offered at universities that are super intriguing and applicable to real world experience that you could be in charge of leading

(BENEFITS OF A PUBLIC HEALTH POLICY MAJOR)

11. LEADERSHIP OPPORTUNITY

Public Health is a world-renowned quality that countries around the world yearn for in many of their departments. There is an ever-growing need for Public Health professionals. For this reason, there is

22. NOT AS DIFFICULT AS STEM

For all of the individuals out there that aren't the keenest on areas of study such as science, engineering and math, Public Health might be the route for you! The courses that the Public Health major requires aren't heavily focused around science and math courses. Although math and science courses to a certain extent are required, they truly are the bare minimum of what can even be categorized as math and science courses!

23. RESEARCH AND PRACTICUM

The great thing about Public Health is that it's a major that truly sees the benefit of research and real-world experience! Typically, as a part of the course work, in order to complete a Public Health bachelor's degree, research and/or practicum experience is required within a course! This provides a great opportunity to not only partake in an educational and applicable to post-grad experience, but it also gets credited towards your degree and course requirement!

24. GREAT OPPORTUNITY FOR PROFESSOR RELATIONSHIPS

As a result of Public Health courses being an extremely "real-life applicable" heavy major, many courses require visits to the Professor's office hours and Professors are usually very conversational when it comes to the course. This is a great perk as Professor relationships really do go a long way when looking at graduate school and even just other future courses that the Professor teaches! Professors have much to offer and it's important that Professors are willing to converse with their students to create clear understanding of their course and Public Health courses provide that perfect opportunity due to the content of the actual course itself!

25. ONLINE OPPORTUNITIES

Public Health courses typically do not require laboratory experience or any courses to that extent. For this reason, many courses that you can take to complete a Public Health major are offered online! This is great for individuals that are trying to balance a full-time work schedule or even just prefer online courses

26. ABILITY TO DOUBLE MAJOR/OR MINOR

The course required for a Public Health major oftentimes also allow for individuals to either double major OR minor in another degree easily! Public Health major requirements typically are not as heavy as other majors and as a result, many students end up having to take "filler courses" to complete the unit graduation requirement! Rather than taking "filler courses," students can easily take courses that go towards either another major or a minor to complement their Public Health major

27. OPPORTUNITY TO STUDY ABROAD

The courses of a Public Health major offer great opportunity to study abroad! Many majors in college do not allow for students to take courses that could satisfy their degree while studying abroad which is why so many students miss the opportunity of studying abroad. Studying abroad is a great opportunity to grow your horizon and ultimately just have the time of your life in a place that you are unfamiliar with! The course load of a Public Health major allows you to do just that

28. FINISH YOUR DEGREE IN FOUR, SOMETIMES THREE, YEARS

If you're wondering if you read that correctly- yep, you did! A Public Health major can be completed in three years sometimes! I was able to go into college with no credits from High School yet still complete my major and minor within three years! There really is no rush, however. Public Health is a major that can easily completed within four years in comparison to some other majors that are assumed five-year graduation majors

29. SUMMER COURSE OPPORTUNITY

Summertime is a great time to utilize to get ahead! However, some majors don't offer many courses over the summer which can make it hard to get ahead over the summertime. The good thing with Public Health courses is that many required courses are offered during the summer! The reason for this being that Public Health courses are more flexible than say some other more strenuous and intense majors which makes a great opportunity for a productive summer

30. DIFFERENT COURSE ROUTES

Above all, Public Health is an amazing major as the course work is not a straight path! There are so many different opportunities and ways to complete certain major specific sections. Rather than just taking a Public Health specific course, as an example, you are able to take an Urban Policy or maybe even an Oceanography course to complete a certain category requirement. Public Health courses are great as there are many different opportunities to explore different courses that aren't specific towards Public Health necessarily

(HOW TO: COMPLETE A PUBLIC HEALTH MAJOR IN 4 YEARS – OR 3)

31. UTILIZE PROFESSOR/TEACHING ASSISTANTS OFFICE HOURS

Ensuring that you are taking advantage of this one-on-one time with your professor or teaching assistant is crucial to succeeding! Sometimes, college lectures can compose of 300 or more students and it's hard for professors to distinguish you amongst a sea of other students. Going in and taking the time to just get to know your professor can help in the long run with not only your understanding of the course, but also that connection with your professor or teaching assistant. They know how to get the best grade in the course which is why it's important to always go in and take the time to ask as many questions as you can

32. ASK ALL OF THE QUESTIONS

To succeed and be on track to graduate with a Public Health major in 4 years, sometimes 3, it's super important that you ask any and all kind of the questions when you are confused about something. Most likely, if you have a question about something, another student is also wondering the same thing so don't be shy! Being confident enough to ask all of the questions that you have will guarantee that you always know everything (or most of) what is being taught! College can get confusing at times as it's meant to be challenging, but doing your part to make sure that you understand everything to the fullest will help you to succeed

33. UTILIZE SUMMER SESSIONS

This is one of the most important tips that I can offer when offering my two cents on how to graduate in 4 years or even earlier! Summer sessions are often seen as time to just blow off and do "nothing" for a couple of months, but while those students sit back and relax, you would be amazed at how ahead others can get if they utilize their time properly during the summer. Public Health major course requirements are typically offered during the summer and can even be taken at a local community college. Use your time wisely as 3 months off can seem enticing to indulge in, but always remember, working hard early to relax later is even more rewarding

34. CONNECT WITH CLASSMATES

When you are surrounded with hundreds of other students that you don't know, this can seem like a daunting task at hand. However, connecting with classmates that are taking the same course as you can be one of the most rewarding things when midterm and final season comes around! Don't forget that college students are all going through the same thing when it comes to college courses. They're HARD! And having your own support system to study with and just ask questions to can be extremely helpful when it comes to acing (or simply passing) a course

35. STAY IN CONTACT WITH YOUR ADVISOR

Advisors can really be the biggest help when it comes to graduating in 4 years or earlier. College courses can be confusing when looking at requirements and seeing what courses should be taken to satisfy certain requirements. There are many requirements and taking even 1 "wrong" course that doesn't satisfy your major requirement can set you back! Figuring out who your advisor is within your major, and staying in contact with them, can help in the long run as they know best and can guide you on the path as to which courses should be taken and help you even create a 4-year plan!

36. MANAGE YOUR TIME

I'm sure time over and over again you've heard that time management is one of the key things when it comes to college. Time management is so important when it comes to college as there are going to be so many things that you are going to be doing at once that it's important to schedule and plan your time out to ensure that everything gets done! You'll be studying, going to classes, engaging in extracurricular activity, studying some more, and even working or doing research. Making sure that you take the time to plan your day and week out will be extremely helpful in succeeding in college

37. GET YOUR SLEEP

Too many students pull all-nighters and although sometimes necessary, it really isn't all that necessary…. Being sleep deprived will affect you in the long run and when you're taking that test, or trying to concentrate on that quiz, you will most definitely feel it. That's why it's so important to ensure that you are sleeping enough as this will ultimately be the most beneficial thing for you and your success in college

38. CREATE GOALS FOR YOURSELF

Goals are the most important thing that will set you apart from others. In no way do you need to create goals in the sense that you have your "whole life planned out," but goals are extremely helpful when it comes to creating a plan for yourself. Create a 4-year goal, then break it down into 1-year goals. Little steps all add up and greatness comes in little, consistent steps

39. UTILIZE A PLANNER

A planner is the best way to manage your time! Whether that means it's a physical planner or a planner/calendar online, use it and stick to it. This will help when you have a million things to do and in the long run it will ease your stress as you'll have your days and weeks planned out! Make sure to regularly update your planner with important exam dates, when to study, and even days that you plan on taking time for yourself! Scheduling your time out will be extremely beneficial in getting things done

40. TAKE TIME FOR YOURSELF!

Getting caught up in college is something that so many students end up having to endure as a result of what seems like an endless amount of work. It's so important that you take time for yourself and give yourself a break to do things you enjoy doing whether then that means future classes will also align for you both which you know you'll have a study buddy for

49. ONLINE GROUPS

As we now live in the digital age, there are many resources online with groups made specifically for the students at your university. Typically these groups can be found on social platforms and they are great resources for: creating group chats with other individuals in the same course as you, asking general questions, and there are even groups for college students to sell items like furniture and books to others that could use it as well!

50. LEARN FROM UPPERCLASSMEN

There are two different ways to learn from mistakes, one being: you do the act and learn from it OR two: you learn from someone else's mistake and avoid having to go through it yourself. Like all things in life, there are smart ways to do something and then there are "other" ways to do it. College is a journey and what best way to learn from then to console in a student above your class level to ensure that you can avoid certain mistakes and save yourself time! Connecting with students older than yourself can be as simple as sparking conversation in lecture with some students around you or connecting with a club that you join

OTHER HELPFUL RESOURCES:

What I Can Do With A Public Health Degree
https://www.worldwidelearn.com/online-education-guide/health-medical/public-health-major.htm

Best Colleges For Public Health
https://www.niche.com/colleges/search/best-colleges-for-public-health/

What Is Public Health
https://www.cdcfoundation.org/what-public-health

READ OTHER

50 THINGS TO KNOW

BOOKS

50 Things to Know

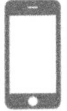

Stay up to date with new releases on Amazon:

https://amzn.to/2VPNGr7